Yoga Foundations

A Beginner's Guide to a Mindful Practice

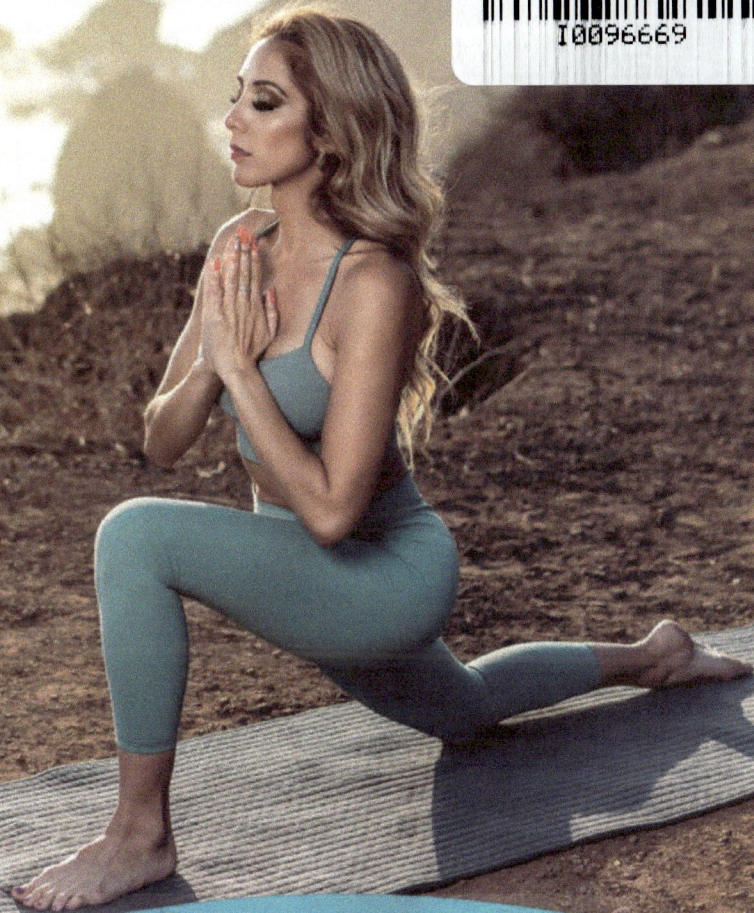

Written by Angelina Jamison
Certified Teacher and Coach

www.yoginiangelina.com

Introduction

Welcome to the transformative world of yoga, where the union of mind, body, and spirit takes center stage in the journey towards holistic well-being. In this ebook, we delve into the myriad benefits that yoga bestows upon both physical and mental health, offering a pathway to balance and vitality.

Yoga, with its ancient roots, has evolved into a modern-day solution for combating the stresses of our fast-paced lives. On a physical level, it enhances flexibility, strength, and posture, which fosters a resilient and agile body. Simultaneously, the practice of yoga extends its profound influence to the realm of mental well-being, promoting relaxation, stress relief, and heightened self-awareness.

As a passionate advocate for yoga and a dedicated teacher, my goal is to share the transformative power of this ancient practice. This ebook serves as a guide to help individuals of all levels embark on their yoga journey, cultivating a deeper connection with themselves and the world around them. My intention is to make the practice accessible and enjoyable, empowering readers to embrace yoga as a lifelong companion on their quest for physical health and mental tranquility. Join me in this exploration, and let yoga become your sanctuary for a balanced and fulfilling life.

Chapters

Chapter 1: Getting Started
- Overview of yoga philosophy and its holistic approach.
- Choosing the right space and time for practice.

Chapter 2: Essential Yoga Poses
- Clear instructions and illustrations for foundational poses (e.g., Mountain Pose, Downward Dog, Warrior Poses).
- Emphasize proper alignment and modifications for beginners.

Chapter 3: Breath Awareness
- Introduction to pranayama (breath control) techniques.
- Guided exercises for deepening breath awareness.

Chapter 4: Mindfulness in Motion
- Explore the connection between movement and mindfulness.
- Tips for cultivating present-moment awareness during yoga practice.

Chapter 5: Building a Routine
- Sample beginner-friendly yoga routines for different time constraints.
- Emphasize consistency and gradual progression.

Chapter 6: Overcoming Challenges
- Address common challenges beginners face and offer solutions.
- Encourage self-compassion and patience.

Chapter 7: Taking Yoga Off the Mat
- Discuss integrating yogic principles into daily life.
- Mindfulness practices for stress relief and improved focus.

Chapter 1

Getting Started

Congratulations on taking the first step towards a journey of self-discovery and well-being through yoga. In this chapter, we lay the groundwork for your practice, exploring the essence of yoga philosophy and providing practical guidance on beginning your transformative journey.

Embracing Yoga Philosophy

Yoga is more than a physical practice; it is a holistic philosophy, that encompasses mind, body, and spirit. Understanding the foundational principles of yoga sets the stage for a meaningful and enriching experience. We'll delve into concepts like unity, breath awareness, and the interconnectedness of all aspects of life.

Creating Your Sacred Space

Your yoga practice extends beyond the mat, and your environment plays a crucial role. Explore the art of creating a sacred space that resonates with tranquility and positivity. Whether it's a corner of your living room or a dedicated room, discover how the right setting can enhance your practice and create a haven for self-reflection.

Timing Your Practice

The rhythm of your day can significantly impact your yoga experience. We'll discuss the optimal times for practice, and considering factors such as energy levels and daily routines. Find a time that aligns with your natural flow, allowing you to fully immerse yourself in the present moment during your practice.

Your Yoga Toolkit

As you embark on your yoga journey, it's essential to have a few basic tools. We'll explore the significance of a quality yoga mat, comfortable attire, and any props that might enhance your practice. Setting yourself up with the right tools ensures comfort and stability during your sessions.

Setting Intentions

Before stepping onto the mat, take a moment to set intentions for your practice. Whether it's cultivating mindfulness, increasing flexibility, or finding inner peace, clarifying your goals adds purpose to each session. We'll discuss the power of intention and how it shapes your journey on and off the mat.

As you delve into the foundational aspects of getting started with yoga, remember that this chapter serves as a guide. Each element is a stepping stone towards a more profound connection with yourself and the practice of yoga. Get ready to embrace the transformative power of this ancient art as you take your first steps on this enriching path.

Chapter 2

Essential Yoga Pose

Welcome to the heart of your yoga practice—exploring essential poses that form the building blocks of a strong and balanced foundation. In this chapter, we will journey through key asanas (poses) with clear instructions and insights, ensuring that your yoga practice is both accessible and transformative.

Mountain Pose (Tadasana)

Begin at the foundation with Mountain Pose, cultivating awareness of alignment, balance, and grounding. This foundational pose sets the tone for many others, teaching you to stand tall with strength and grace.

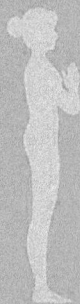

Downward-Facing Dog (Adho Mukha Svanasana)

Explore the invigorating Downward-Facing Dog, promoting flexibility in the spine, shoulders, and hamstrings. This pose is a cornerstone, linking movement with breath, and providing a rejuvenating stretch.

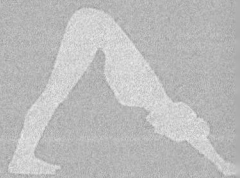

Warrior Poses (Virabhadrasana I, II, and III)

Introduce strength and stability through the Warrior series. These poses build resilience and focus while engaging major muscle groups, promoting both physical and mental endurance.

Tree Pose (Vrksasana)

Find your balance in Tree Pose, a graceful pose that enhances concentration and stability. As you root down through one leg and extend through the spine, experience a beautiful blend of strength and serenity.

Child's Pose (Balasana)

Discover the restorative power of Child's Pose —a gentle resting posture that provides a moment of reprieve. This pose encourages surrender and introspection, making it an essential part of any yoga sequence.

Cobra Pose (Bhujangasana)

Open your heart and strengthen your back with Cobra Pose. This backbend promotes flexibility in the spine while toning the muscles of the back, awakening a sense of vitality.

Seated Forward Bend (Paschimottanasana)

Cultivate flexibility in the spine and hamstrings through the Seated Forward Bend. This pose encourages forward folding, promoting relaxation and calming the nervous system.

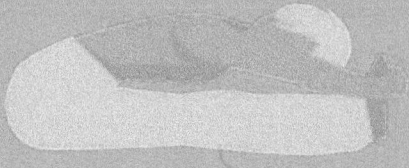

Corpse Pose (Savasana)

Conclude your practice with Corpse Pose, a posture of deep relaxation. Savasana allows your body and mind to absorb the benefits of your practice, leaving you with a sense of tranquility and rejuvenation.

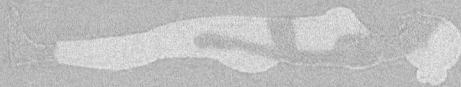

Chapter 3

Breath Awareness

In the rhythmic dance of yoga, the breath is your ever-present partner. This chapter explores the profound connection between breath and movement, introducing you to the art of pranayama—breath control. Let's dive into the transformative power of conscious breathing and discover how it can enhance your overall well-being.

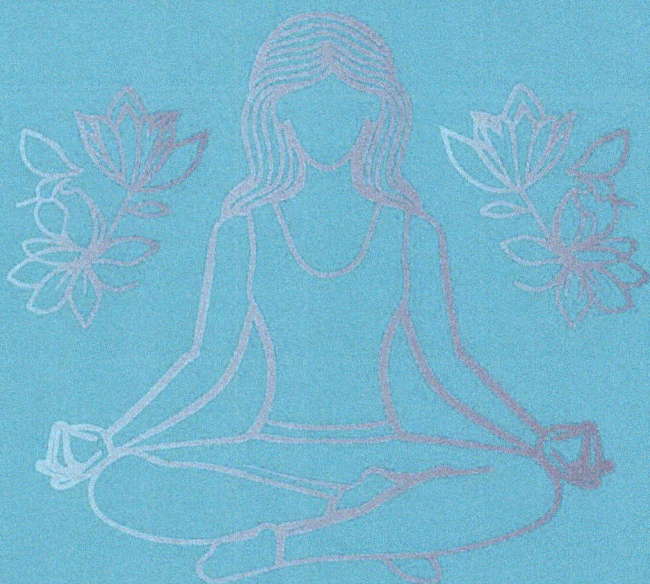

The Breath-Mind Connection

Begin by understanding the intimate relationship between breath and the mind. Explore how the quality of your breath influences your mental state, and vice versa. This awareness forms the foundation for harnessing the full potential of your breath in yoga.

Ujjayi Breath

Enter the world of Ujjayi breath, a deep, oceanic breath that not only anchors your practice but also calms the nervous system. Learn the technique of engaging the throat to create a subtle, soothing sound, providing a steady rhythm to guide your movements.

Dirga Pranayama (Three-Part Breath)

Explore the Three-Part Breath to expand lung capacity and increase oxygen intake. This foundational breathing technique involves consciously directing the breath into different areas of the lungs, promoting a sense of fullness and vitality.

Nadi Shodhana (Alternate Nostril Breathing)

Discover balance and harmony through Nadi Shodhana, a pranayama technique that involves alternating breath between the nostrils. This practice not only brings equilibrium to the left and right hemispheres of the brain but also fosters a deep sense of calm.

Breath Awareness in Asanas

Integrate breath awareness into your yoga poses, synchronizing movement with the inhalations and exhalations Explore how conscious breathing enhances your connection to the present moment and deepens the benefits of each posture.

*Pranayama for Relaxation

Unwind and release tension through pranayama techniques specifically designed for relaxation. Dive into practices like Bhramari (Bee Breath) and Shitali (Cooling Breath) to soothe the nervous system and promote a tranquil state of mind.

Breath and Meditation

Experience the transformative synergy of breath and meditation. Learn techniques to focus your attention in the breath, fostering a sense of inner stillness and mindfulness. Discover how the breath becomes a gateway to a quieter, more centered mind.

As you delve into the realm of breath awareness, remember that your breath is a constant companion, guiding you through the ebb and flow of your yoga practice. Embrace the power of conscious breathing as a source of vitality, presence, and inner harmony.

Chapter 4

Mindfulness in Motion

Welcome to the heart of yogic practice, where movement becomes a mindful exploration of the self. In this chapter, we delve into the art of moving with intention, fostering a deep connection between mind and body. Prepare to embark on a journey of mindfulness in motion.

Cultivating Present-Moment Awareness

Mindfulness in yoga begins with being fully present in each moment. Explore techniques to anchor your attention to the sensations of the body, the rhythm of your breath, and the unfolding of each movement. As you cultivate awareness, witness the transformative power of being fully engaged in the now.

Moving Meditation

Discover the concept of moving meditation, where each pose becomes a dynamic expression of mindfulness. Explore how intentional movement can quiet the mind, offering a respite from the demands of daily life. As you flow through your practice, let the movements be a meditation in motion.

Mindful Transitions Between Poses

The space between poses is as crucial as the poses themselves. Learn to navigate these transitions with grace and awareness. Mindful movements between poses not only enhance the fluidity of your practice but also deepen your connection to the breath.

Listening to Your Body

Your body is a wise guide on this yogic journey. Explore the practice of embodied mindfulness, where you learn to listen to the subtle cues your body provides. By tuning in to sensations, you cultivate a compassionate understanding of your body's needs and limitations.

Focus on Alignment

Mindful movement includes a keen awareness of alignment. Dive into the details of proper alignment for various poses, understanding how alignment contributes to both the effectiveness and safety of your practice. Aligning mind and body creates a harmonious balance.

Integrating Mindfulness into Daily Activities

Extend the principles of mindfulness beyond the mat. Explore how the mindfulness cultivated in yoga can be applied to daily activities, fostering a sense of presence and purpose in every moment. Your yoga practice becomes a catalyst for a more mindful and fulfilling life.

Breath as Your Anchor

Throughout your mindful practice, the breath remains a steadfast anchor. Explore how the rhythmic flow of breath grounds you in the present moment, serving as a guide through each pose and transition. The breath becomes a constant reminder to stay connected and centered.

As you engage in mindfulness in motion, allow each movement to be an opportunity for self-discovery. Embrace the transformative power of moving with intention, and witness the profound integration of mind, body, and spirit in your yoga practice.

Chapter 5

Building a Routine

Congratulations on reaching a pivotal point in your yoga journey. In this chapter, we shift our focus to the construction of a balanced and sustainable yoga routine. Whether you have a few minutes or an hour, creating a consistent practice empowers you to reap the full benefits of yoga in your daily life.

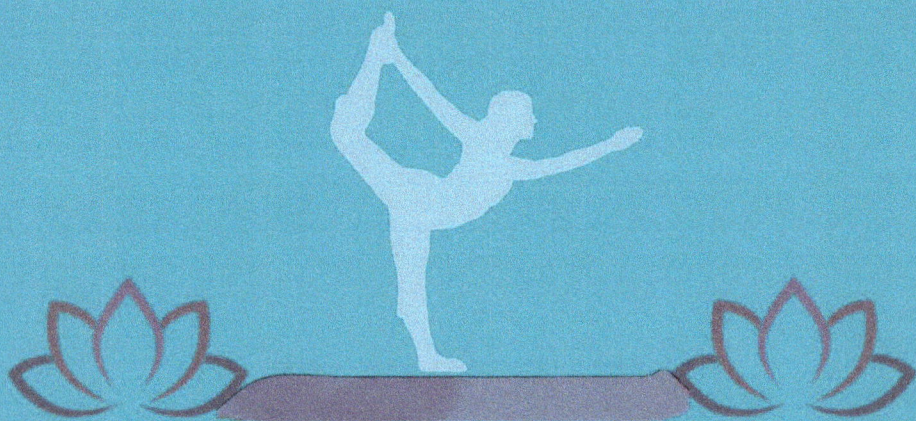

Setting Realistic Goals

Begin by defining your yoga goals, whether they involve enhancing flexibility, building strength, or finding moments of peace. Setting realistic and achievable goals forms the foundation for a purposeful and fulfilling practice.

Tailoring Your Practice to Your Schedule

Explore how to adapt your yoga routine to fit your schedule. Whether you have 10 minutes or an hour, discover flexible sequences and modifications that allow you to integrate yoga seamlessly into your daily life.

Morning and Evening Practices
Delve into the benefits of morning and evening yoga practices. Morning sessions can invigorate and prepare you for the day ahead, while evening practices offer a soothing transition from the busyness of life to a state of relaxation.

Creating a Well-Rounded Sequence
Craft a well-rounded yoga sequence that addresses different aspects of your well-being. Incorporate warm-up poses, a variety of postures, breathwork, and a final relaxation to ensure a comprehensive and holistic practice.

Consistency Over Intensity
Emphasize the importance of consistency in your yoga routine. Regular, mindful practice yields more significant benefits than sporadic intense sessions. Discover the power of small, daily commitments to foster lasting positive change.

Gradual Progression
Approach your yoga routine with a mindset of gradual progression. As you become more comfortable with certain poses, consider adding variations or exploring more advanced postures. Allow your practice to evolve organically over time

Contrary to popular belief pain is *not* gain.

Combining Yoga Styles

Explore the richness of yoga by combining different styles within your routine. Whether it's Hatha, Vinyasa, or Restorative, integrating diverse practices provides a well-rounded experience, addressing various physical and mental needs.

Self-Reflection and Adaptation

Regularly reflect on your yoga journey. Notice how your body and mind respond to different practices. Be open to adapting your routine based on your evolving needs and goals, ensuring that your yoga practice remains a dynamic and personalized experience.

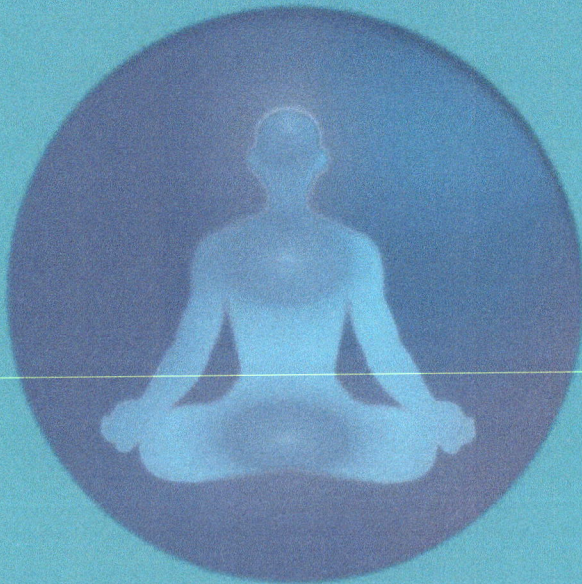

As you build your yoga routine, remember that it is a dynamic and personal journey. Tailor your practice to suit your lifestyle, embrace consistency, and allow your routine to be a source of joy, vitality, and self-discovery. Your yoga mat becomes a sacred space for growth and well-being.

Chapter 6

Overcoming Challenges

Embarking on a yoga journey is a rewarding endeavor, but like any worthwhile pursuit, it comes with its own set of challenges. In this chapter, we address common obstacles that beginners often encounter and provide guidance on how to navigate them, fostering resilience and a deeper connection with your practice.

Embracing the Learning Curve

One of the initial challenges is grappling with the learning curve of yoga postures, breathwork, and philosophy. Understand that it's perfectly normal to feel uncertain or uncomfortable at first. Embrace the learning process, be patient with yourself, and celebrate small victories along the way.

Patience as a Virtue

Patience is a cornerstone of yoga. Whether you're working on mastering a challenging pose or progressing in your mindfulness practice, recognize that growth takes time. Develop a patient mindset, understanding that each step forward, no matter how small, contributes to your overall journey.

Navigating Physical Limitations

Physical limitations can be a hurdle, but they need not be roadblocks. Yoga is about adaptation and modification. Explore variations of poses that suit your body's needs, and focus on the essence of each posture rather than perfection. Gradual progress is a testament to your dedication.

Balancing Effort and Ease

Finding the right balance between effort and ease in yoga is an ongoing challenge. Avoid pushing yourself too hard, yet don't shy away from challenges. Learning to listen to your body and finding the equilibrium between pushing boundaries and respecting limitations is a valuable skill.

Quietening the Mind

Quieting the mind during yoga can be challenging, especially in a world filled with distractions. Acknowledge that the mind's tendency to wander is part of the practice. Use breath awareness and mindfulness techniques to gently bring your focus back to the present moment, fostering a calmer mind over time.

Consistency Amidst Busy Lives

Maintaining a consistent practice amidst the demands of a busy life is a common struggle. Establishing a routine that fits your schedule, even if it's brief, creates a foundation for consistency. To reiterate its importance, regular, shorter sessions are often more beneficial than sporadic, intense practices.

Building Mental Resilience

Yoga is not just about physical resilience but also mental resilience. Face challenges with a positive mindset, viewing them as opportunities for growth. Develop mental strength through breathwork, meditation, and cultivating a present-moment awareness that extends beyond the mat.

Embracing Self-Compassion

Above all, embrace self-compassion on your yoga journey. Acknowledge that challenges are part of the process, and perfection is not the goal. Treat yourself with kindness, especially when facing difficulties. A compassionate approach to your practice fosters a more nurturing and sustainable yoga journey.

Remember, the challenges you encounter on your yoga journey are not so much roadblocks as they are stepping stones. Each obstacle is an opportunity for growth, self-discovery, and a deeper connection with the transformative power of yoga. Approach challenges with an open heart and a resilient spirit, knowing that overcoming them is an integral part of the beautiful journey you've embarked upon.

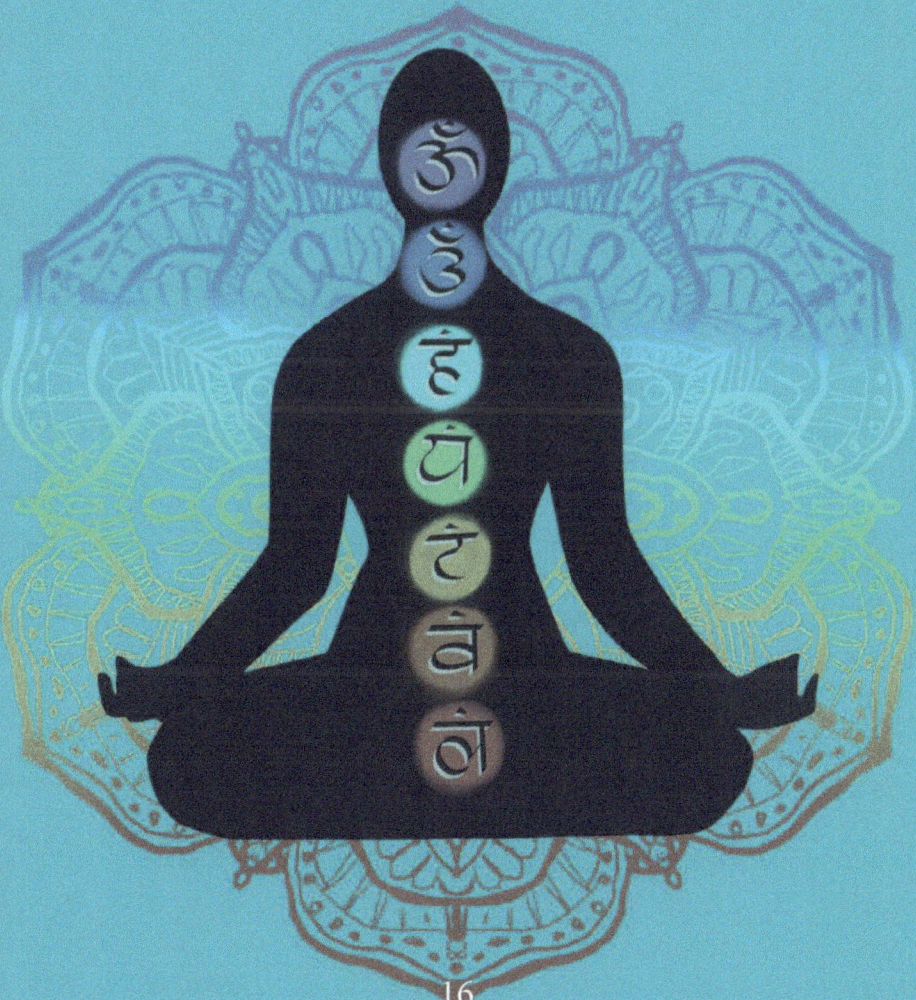

Chapter 7

Taking Yoga Off the Mat

As your yoga practice blossoms, it becomes a powerful tool for holistic well-being beyond the confines of the mat. In this chapter, we explore how the principles and mindfulness cultivated during yoga can be seamlessly integrated into your daily life, creating a harmonious and balanced existence.

Mindful Living Beyond Asanas

Yoga extends far beyond physical postures. Embrace yoga as a way of life by incorporating mindfulness into everyday activities. Whether you're walking, eating, or working, carry the awareness and intention cultivated on the mat into each moment.

Stress Reduction Techniques

Explore practical stress reduction techniques derived from yoga philosophy. Incorporate breathwork, meditation, and mindfulness practices into your daily routine to navigate stressors with grace and resilience.

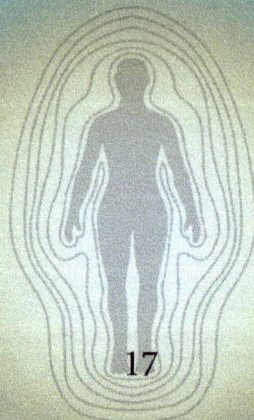

Mindful Eating

Transform your relationship with food through mindful eating. Bring awareness to the textures, flavors, and sensations during meals. This practice not only enhances digestion but also cultivates gratitude for the nourishment your body receives.

Mindful Communication

Yoga teaches us to listen—to our bodies, our breath, and our surroundings. Extend this attentive listening to your interactions with others. Practice mindful communication by being present, empathetic, and fully engaged in conversations.

Cultivating Gratitude

Gratitude is a cornerstone of a fulfilled life. Take moments each day to reflect on the aspects of your life for which you are grateful. This simple practice enhances both a positive mindset and your overall sense of well-being.

Finding Stillness Amidst Chaos

In the midst of a fast-paced world, discover the art of finding stillness within. Through brief moments of meditation or mindful pauses, you can create islands of calm amidst the chaos, fostering mental clarity and resilience.

Acts of Kindness and Compassion

Yoga encourages kindness and compassion towards oneself and others. Extend this compassion beyond the mat by incorporating acts of kindness into your daily life. Small gestures ripple outward, creating a positive impact on your surroundings.

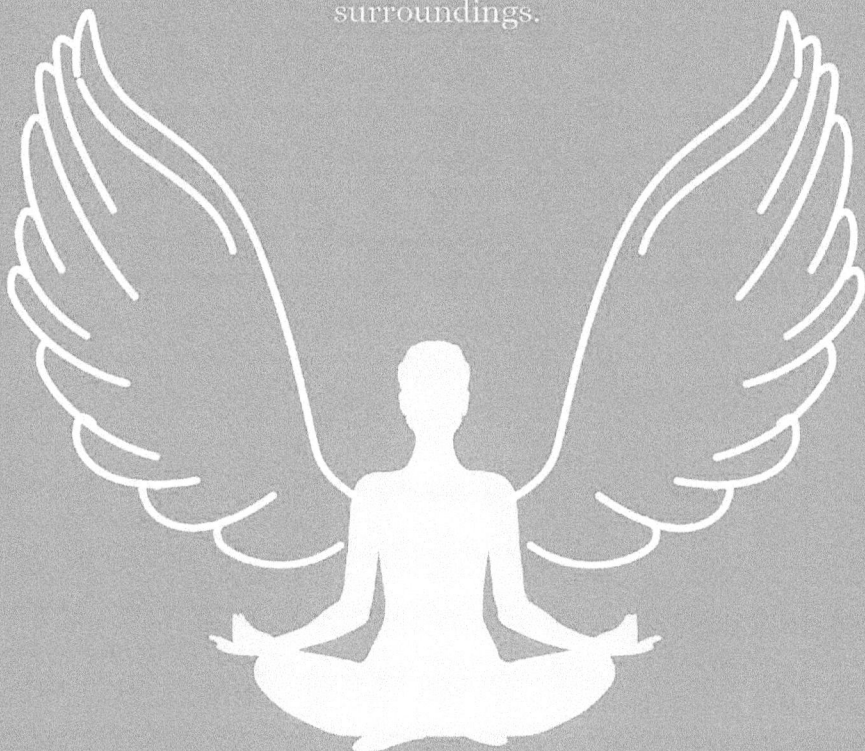

Reflecting on Your Journey

Regularly reflect on your yoga journey and its impact on your life. Consider how your practice has influenced your mindset, habits, and relationships. Recognize the growth and positive changes that have unfolded, nurturing a sense of gratitude and self-awareness.

As you embrace yoga off the mat, you'll discover that the transformative power of this ancient practice extends far beyond the physical. It becomes a guiding philosophy for living with intention, mindfulness, and compassion a blueprint for a balanced and purposeful life.

Resources

Books
"The Heart of Yoga: Developing a Personal Practice"
by T.K.V. Desikachar

"Light on Yoga" by B.K.S. Iyengar
- "The Key Muscles of Yoga" by Ray Long

Online Courses
Yoga Alliance (yogaalliance.org)
Offers a variety of online courses for both beginners and
experienced practitioners, covering different styles and
aspects of yoga.

Mobile Apps
YogaGlo: Provides a vast library of online yoga classes with
different durations and styles.

Insight Timer: Offers a diverse range of guided meditations,
including those focused on mindfulness and breath
awareness.

Podcasts
"The Yoga Podcast" by Karen O'Donnell Clarke:
Explores various aspects of yoga, from philosophy to
practical tips for enhancing your practice.

Yoga Journals and Magazines
"Yoga Journal" and "Yoga International"
Both publications provide articles, tutorials, and insights
into different aspects of yoga, including poses, philosophy,
and lifestyle.

Resources Cont...

Local Yoga Workshops and Retreats
Attend workshops or retreats led by experienced yoga teachers in your community or explore opportunities in yoga retreat destinations. These immersive experiences can deepen your practice and offer a fresh perspective.

Yoga Communities and Forums
Engage with online yoga communities and forums, such as Reddit's r/yoga or specialized Facebook groups. Participating in discussions and sharing experiences with fellow practitioners can provide valuable insights and recommendations for further learn

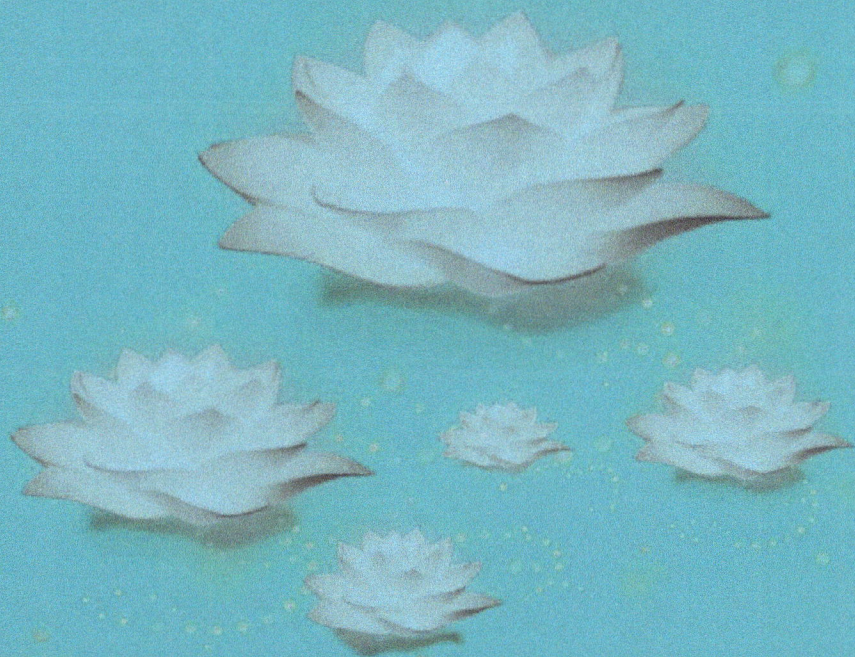

Resources Cont...

Website:
www.yoginiangelina.com

YouTube:
www.youtube.com/@YoginiAngelina

Instagram:
www.instagram.com/yoginiangelina

Cover Photo Credits:
Revo Media

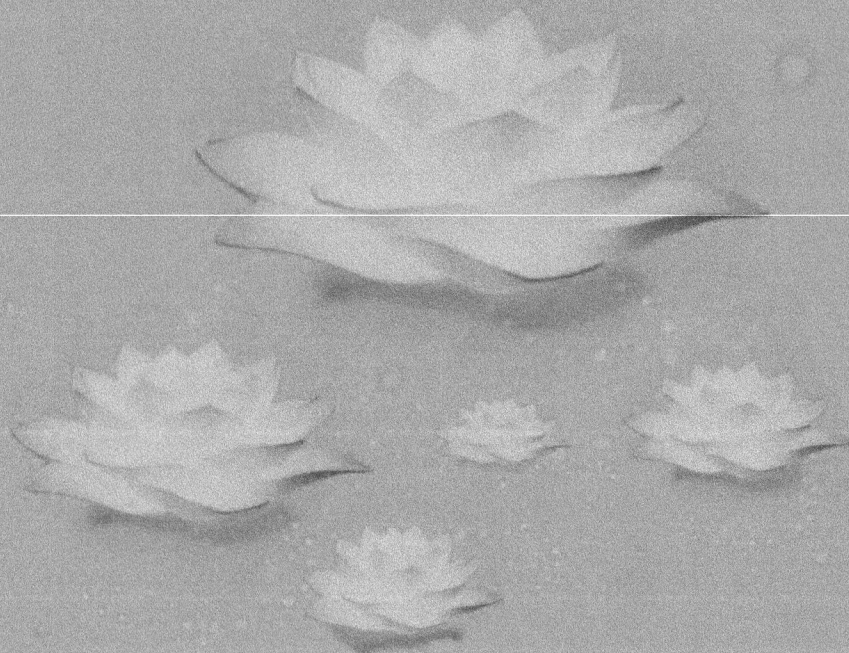

Healing is a process and it's something that doesn't happen overnight. "It takes time. It takes patience. It takes perseverance. It also takes determination. Most of all, it takes a whole lot of self love."

"OWNING OUR STORY CAN BE HARD BUT NOT NEARLY AS DIFFICULT AS SPENDING OUR LIVES RUNNING FROM IT."

~ Angelina Jamison ~

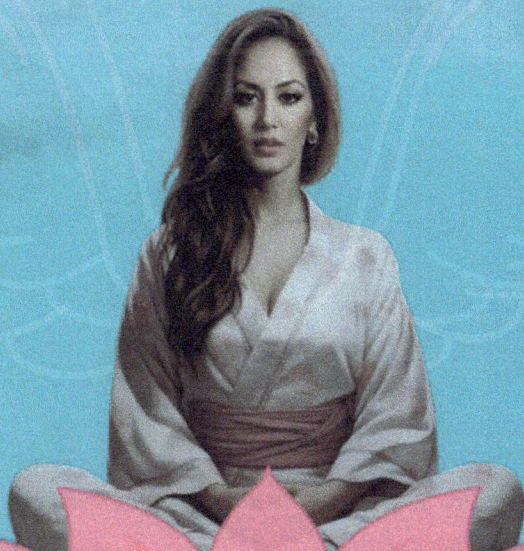

About the author

Angelina Jamison

Empowering Souls Through Yoga and Digital
Marketing

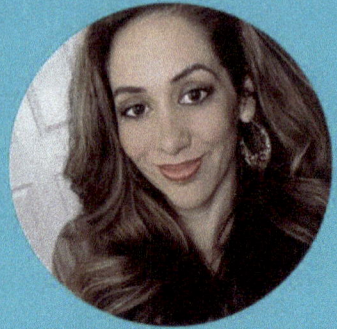

A visionary with a heart dedicated to
empowerment, Angelina has spent the last 16
years transforming lives as a yoga meditation
instructor. Her journey began on the mat,
where she discovered the profound impact of
inner evolution on overall well-being.

Born with a passion for guiding individuals toward self-discovery, Angelina
has become a beacon of light for those seeking balance and fulfillment. As a
yoga meditation instructor, she has shared the transformative power of
mindfulness, teaching not only physical postures but also the healing
benefits of meditation. Her classes are not just about stretching the body
but nurturing the soul, understanding that true evolution starts from the
inside out.

In a world marked by constant change, Angelina recognized the growing
importance of digital presence and marketing. Driven by her mission to
reach and empower more people, she embarked on a new journey to blend
ancient wisdom with modern strategies. Angelina is on a mission to
democratize the digital landscape, helping as many individuals as possible
start their digital marketing journeys.
Angelina's expertise lies in bridging the gap between spirituality and
technology, creating a holistic approach to personal and financial growth.
Through her guidance, motivated individuals are empowered to build
passive streams of income, unlocking new possibilities and financial
freedom.

Her unique perspective stems from years of understanding the
interconnectedness of mind, body, and digital presence. Angelina's
commitment goes beyond traditional boundaries, and she strives to create a
community where self-discovery meets entrepreneurial spirit.

In the ever-evolving landscape of self-improvement and online
entrepreneurship, Angelina stands as a trailblazer, inspiring others to
embrace both the ancient wisdom of yoga meditation and the modern
opportunities presented by digital marketing. Her journey is a testament to
the transformative power of holistic growth, proving that by aligning mind,
body, and business, individuals can achieve a life of purpose, abundance,
and balance.

www.ingramcontent.com/pod-product-compliance
Lightning Source LLC
Chambersburg PA
CBHW052026030426
42335CB00026B/3305